Today's Private Practice

Strategies for Building a Thriving Managed-Care Free Psychotherapy Practice

By William D. Morgan, Psy.D.

Here's What People Are Saying About "Today's Private Practice"

"In 'Today's Private Practice,' Dr. Bill Morgan has created a simple, practical, clinician-friendly formula to achieve success as a solo practitioner. I wish this book had been available when I was getting started!"

— Lisa Kramer, MSW, PCC, life coach and coach trainer, president of Living with Intention

"This excellent guide is loaded with empowering advice and strategies to help any therapist take his or her practice to the next level. Even though I have worked outside of managed care for many years, I now see many exciting opportunities that exist for me that I never before realized were possible. In one single source, Dr. Morgan gives you all you need to know to make your practice explode with new clients and opportunities."

— Jeffrey Bernstein, Ph.D. Licensed Psychologist in Private Practice and author of "Why Can't You Read My Mind?"

"As therapists, we have a great deal to offer the world. This book gives readers a very straightforward, unapologetic approach to telling the community about their services. Even the most uncertain reader will feel emboldened to take these steps to improve their practice."

— Ari Tuckman, Psy.D., Licensed Psychologist

"Dr. Morgan's book is perfect for new and veteran therapists who are building their practices. Dr. Morgan breaks down difficult concepts in a very friendly, conversational tone that every therapy practitioner will be able to relate to."

— Jeffrey Kaplan, Ph.D., Psychologist, President, Interpersonal Growth Workshops Inc.

Dear Reader,

Congratulations! You hold in your hands the limited first edition of "Today's Private Practice: Strategies for Building a Thriving Managed-Care Free Psychotherapy Practice."

By being one of a select group to purchase this book, you have early access to concepts that are changing the lives of psychologists and mental health professionals.

After close to two decades in the profession, I am convinced these pages represent key concepts for struggling practioners.

Send along your suggestions, critiques and stories. With your contributions, this book will evolve into an even more helpful one.

Sincerely,

Bill Morgan

TODAY'S PRIVATE PRACTICE: STRATEGIES FOR BUILDING A THRIVING MANAGED-CARE FREE PSYCHOTHERAPY PRACTICE

by William D. Morgan, Psy.D.

Published by:

Golden Hill Publishing

513 Howell Lane, Havertown, PA 19083

Printed in the United States of America by:

Morris Publishing

3212 East Highway 30, P.O. Box 2110, Kearney, NE 68847

800-650-7888 / www.morrispublishing.com

ISBN: 978-0-9773577-0-3

Library of Congress Control Number: 2005910139

First Printing January 2006

For information contact:

William D. Morgan, Psy.D.

63 Chestnut Road, Paoli, PA 19301

Info@TodaysPrivatePractice.com / 610-687-7695

Editing & Book Design:

Jack Out of the Box Designs

www.jackoutofthebox.com

CONTENTS

Introduction **1**

Chapter 1 - Foundational Concepts **5**

Why Are Your Reading This Book?
Why I Wrote This Book
The Current Situation In the Psychotherapy Marketplace
The Fundamental Strategy
N+P+F=Success
Are You Ready to Break Free of Managed Care?

Chapter 2 - Getting Clients **19**

Marketing
Choosing a Niche Market
Developing a Service Line
Multiple Streams of Referrals
The Marketing Cycle
Marketing and Who You Are
Get Out of the Office
Developing a Plan
12 Marketing Ideas to Build Your Practice That You Can Implement Right Away

Chapter 3 - The Eight Steps **43**

1. Find a Niche
2. Discover the Niche Market's Problems
3. Develop Solutions
4. Design Packaging
5. Develop a Marketing Plan
6. Implement Marketing
7. Create a Follow-Up System
8. Keep It Going and Growing

Chapter 4 - Streams of Psychotherapy Income 55
- Traditional Services
- Getting Published
- Teaching
- E-books
- E-courses
- Personal Coaching
- Live Workshops, Retreats, Trainings
- TeleSeminars
- Consulting
- Forensic Consulting
- Web sites
- Licensing Programs
- Training Other Professionals

Chapter 5 - Transitioning 79
- The Key Concepts
- Vision
- The Business of Private Practice
- Money
- Beef Up Your Systems
- Therapists, Take Your Own Medicine — Work On Yourself

Conclusion 89
- Are you Ready?
- Introduction to the Today's Private Practice Membership Web Site, www.TodaysPrivatePractice.com

Appendices 93
- A Working List of Niche Markets
- A Working List of Personal Growth/Skills Building Areas of Felt Need
- A Working List of Traditional (And Some Non-Traditional) Services Not Covered By Managed Care

About the Author 99

Get In Touch 101

Acknowledgements 103

INTRODUCTION

As you will soon find in the following pages, I believe it is possible to help people and make a good living while enjoying an enviable lifestyle.

Today a mental health practitioner in private practice faces this choice: Either work under contract for a profit-driven managed-care company and accept whatever fees and conditions they decree, or find clients who are willing to pay out of pocket for high-quality services.

Yes, you can decide to operate primarily outside of managed care.

I have, and so have hundreds, maybe thousands, of therapists.

To do this, you need more than a bunch of tips and techniques. You need a systematized approach that works and some necessary skill sets.

That's what this book and companion web site, www.TodaysPrivatePractice.com, are all about.

This book is written with the mental health or psychology professional — psychologists, psychiatrists, social workers, counselors, marriage and family therapists and others — in mind.

But, the concepts apply to professionals of many human service professions, such as dentists, physicians, personal coaches, chiropractors, massage therapists and physical therapists.

Too often practitioners attend a workshop or read a book, get a lot of ideas and learn techniques, but then struggle to successfully implement them. They may eventually give up, due to the lack of results, and think, "It's not for me."

The Today's Private Practice approach is different. We provide the tools, structure and support you need. It is an immensely practical system that can be customized to who you are.

Today's Private Practice was created out of the realization that many therapists have doubts about the viability of the dream they once had of a practice where they help people and are well paid.

CHAPTER 1 —

FOUNDATIONAL CONCEPTS

Why Are You Reading This Book?

Maybe you are tired of working in the managed-care system and are thinking about starting a managed-care free practice.

Maybe you have started a private practice, but are struggling to get private-pay clients.

Maybe you have a good private practice, but feel you have not realized your full potential. You want a full practice of well-paying clients.

Maybe you just want a few great ideas to take your practice to the next level. One good idea can sometimes make a big difference.

Private practice has changed drastically from what it was a little over a decade ago and continues to evolve. Much of the change has been related to the expansion of managed-care insurance.

Many practitioners have been able to thrive while others struggle. Many psychologists and other professionals have left private practice, unable to successfully adapt.

Some of the concerns and frustrations I hear expressed include:

- Low fees
- Being undervalued in the managed-care system
- Lower quality of services in the managed-care system
- Discouragement with the lowered income, additional strains and burdens
- Managed care is too much in the driver's seat
- Encountered inequities in the managed-care system
- Ethical dilemmas about such things as continuity of care and terminating therapy too soon
- Having to work too many hours to make ends meet
- Time-consuming authorization, billing and administrative work
- A pervasive current of gloom regarding the future of the profession

Perhaps you, like many professionals I talk to in the consulting and coaching part of my work, aspire toward a more rewarding and lucrative practice.

That's where I was several years ago.

As a practicing psychologist, I know what you are likely experiencing. I love being a psychologist in private practice, but also understand how challenging it can be.

I also know how to make a practice grow and stay successful. And, I can show you what it takes to earn a good income completely outside of managed care.

Over the years, I have created a practice that provides me and my clients high levels of satisfaction. And, I can show you how to do that, too.

Some of you, especially Charter Members of the Today's Private Practice monthly membership, have already begun this journey. You have begun to implement the mindset and practical how-to steps behind the Today's Private Practice school of thought. Maybe you work with a business coach or are part of a group of practitioners dialoging about practice-building.

I foresee that more and more practitioners will discover financial success in private practice outside of managed care. These practitioners will increase their satisfaction level and sustain it.

Today's Private Practice is about a model of consistently making a difference in people's lives, and sustaining success and satisfaction as a professional.

Fee-for-service private practice is not dying, but it is changing.

While many practices are struggling, others are thriving. Successful practitioners have figured out how to promote their services effectively, and you can too.

While many successful therapists learned how to grow their practice by trial and error, you can save months or years by utilizing the Today's Private Practice approach.

Why I Wrote This Book

I have two purposes in writing this book. First, I want to share that transitioning to a full fee-for-service practice is quite possible. Second, I want to help you create and realize your vision for a satisfying and successful career.

Vision is important, and we deal with it in detail later in this book. Transitioning to a thriving practice will also require determination and follow-through.

I've divided the book into several major sections.

In the first section, I talk generally about the philosophy behind the shift to setting up a managed-care free practice. I talk about the general formula for attracting private pay clients and the opportunities it creates.

In the second section, I invite you to explore a different view of marketing. Getting private-pay clients is a stress point for many practitioners, and a topic with which many are not comfortable or skilled. As we look at marketing in a fresh way, I hope you will see that there are simple, effective ways you can build your practice — and enjoy doing it.

In section three, I outline an eight-step approach to implementing the Today's Private Practice model in your practice.

In the fourth section, I outline practical applications of the approach to developing multiple streams of referrals and income. In every stream, there are opportunities to transfer the science and art we've learned.

In section five, I address the transition from where you are now to where you want to be. I share strategies to help ease the transition to a successful practice.

This book is not a textbook or cookbook on building a private practice. Rather, in an informal, down-to-earth, no-fluff approach to the subject, I hope it conveys intriguing, helpful and practical strategies for how therapists can see greater success and satisfaction in their careers and businesses.

Keep reading to find out how to get more out of your profession — personally and financially.

The Current Situation in the Psychotherapy Marketplace

Let's face it, private practice has changed from what it was 10 to 15 years ago. Managed care has made therapeutic services more accessible to the masses, but also lowered standards of service and diminished the perceived value of therapy. Providers receive less compensation, have more administrative work and feel less in control of the service they provide.

My Own Story

I completed my master's degree in counseling psychology in 1988 and began practicing as a counselor in a private group practice. Managed care had not yet surfaced in the metropolitan area where I was located. Things went well. I returned to graduate school in 1992 while continuing to practice, with the vision of obtaining my doctorate in clinical psychology and a more lucrative and independent practice as a licensed psychologist. Shortly after beginning my doctoral degree program, managed care was taking over the market in our area and across the nation.

As the impact was becoming plain, I remember the dismay of my fellow classmates who wondered if they were going to be able to earn enough as a psychologist to repay their student loans. I heard stories of practitioners leaving private practice to join groups doing managed-care work because they could not make it work in the traditional private practice model. Some were even leaving the profession.

After completing my training and obtaining my doctorate and license, I worked in a large managed-care driven group. The pay was low; I received about half of the fees collected from managed-care insurance, which was paying about half of the going rate in our area for psychologist fees. There were numerous problems and frustrations dealing with managed-care companies. I had to work long hours and many evenings to support my family.

Finally, after much deliberation and inspiration from practitioners who were successful in managed-care-free practices, I decided to go out on a limb and set up my own private office. From the outset, I established a private-pay-only practice. I did this for several reasons:

- I believe that managed care does not cover high quality services
- Clients want and deserve customized attention
- Many people value real privacy, which they cannot have in managed care
- I believe I deserve to make a good living in the profession, and can design a more satisfying workplace outside of managed care

The question was, would enough people be willing to pay out of pocket for services?

The answer was and is YES.

More and more, people are coming to the realization that insurance no longer covers high-quality therapy. If people desire it, they have to pay out of pocket. If people pay less, they get less.

I researched what it takes to set up a successful private practice. I worked with a business coach to guide me in areas in which I was unfamiliar (what they don't teach you in graduate school).

And now at the other end of the transition, I can say it was one of the best things I ever did.

The Fundamental Strategy

The thing is, you can make a living helping others. But you have to let go of the idea that the traditional way is the only way.

Psychotherapists can leverage their talents, expertise and abilities in many ways. There are many possible formats for delivering psychological help.

So, how do you, as a therapist, format what you have to offer? To begin, try looking at your services as a solution to a specific problem rather than as treatment for an illness.

In the traditional model, clients must be ill. In order for people to access their health insurance, they must be diagnosed as having a mental illness. This is the medical model.

This creates a barrier for many people to choose to utilize psychological services. They do not want to see themselves as mentally ill and in need of treatment. But, as we shall see, even healthy, high-functioning individuals can benefit from psychological services.

Thus, we tremendously expand our potential market when we reduce the stigma of utilizing our services and focus less on pathology.

Instead, we may adopt a problem-solving/skill-building model, in which clients no longer need to be ill to use our services and receive benefit.

Psychology is not just for the sick.

For example, Martin Seligman's book "Authentic Happiness" (2002) and Daniel Goleman's books "Emotional Intelligence" (1995) and "Working with Emotional Intelligence" (1998) provide us with frameworks we can use in a problem-solving/skill-building model. See also Reivich and Shatté's (2002) "The Resilience Factor." Rather than focus on illness and therapy, we can talk about increasing personal and career effectiveness, personal growth, increasing life satisfaction and resiliency.

Can you see how this broadens the reach and impact of our services? We can provide solutions to life's problems and challenges, without the stigma of a diagnosis — keeping in mind that there is certainly a place for traditional services and therapy for mental illness for those that need it.

In this non-traditional approach, we seek to use our services to:

1. Answer a specific problem or challenge
2. Target a service toward a specific group of people
3. Utilize a tangible format.

So, whether you intend to use traditional therapy as 25 percent or 75 percent of your practice pie, it's a smart move to identify what non-traditional services you could add to the mix of streams of income for yourself. Read on.

N + P + F = SUCCESS

There are three steps to developing a psychology-based, non-traditional service line that will have great value and impact.

The simple three-step formula to creating a new income-producing service is:

Niche + Problem + Format = Service

If your mission is to positively impact other people, this formula will do it. Let's look more closely.

1. Pick a Niche Market.

It could be divorced parents, ACOA Adults, breast-cancer patients, ADHD executives, children of divorce, attorneys, clergy swamped with congregational people problems or smokers who want to quit.

You can take your services to the workplace and target stressed workers, downsizing companies, businesses in change or troubled employees and departments.

Many more possibilities are listed later in this book.

2. Identify a specific problem or challenge that's happening in that niche market.

It could be managing stress, self-management, conflict, interpersonal skills, changing culture within a company, work-life balance, co-parenting or dissatisfaction with life, relationships or career.

There's a multitude of possibilities.

3. Choose the format to deliver your solution.

This is the packaging that your solution will come in.

Example:

Niche: Divorced parents

Problem: Collaboration with ex on parenting; high conflict in communication

Format: 10 co-parenting sessions organized around a five-step process

Equals: A marketable income stream

Ask yourself: For what services will people feel a need and be willing to pay for out of pocket?

Are You Ready to Break Free of Managed Care?

Managed care does not cover high-quality therapy or many psychologically based services for which people feel a need. People will pay for services they perceive as a sufficient value to themselves.

The value of private-pay services over managed-care services are that they are more personalized, remove the stigma of the medical model and clinic setting, offer true privacy and are more effective.

In addition, we have the distinction and opportunity to offer services from a personal growth model in addition to or in place of the traditional medical model.

When you let go of managed care, you:

1. Assume control of your services, income and lifestyle.

There is greater opportunity for financial success and satisfaction in your work.

2. Have greater enjoyment and passion for your work.

You won't be as bored with your work, and will be less susceptible to burnout. This model encourages you to do more of the work that taps into who you are, what you love to do and unleashes your creativity. You will have greater variety in the work you do, not the same basic work day-in and day-out.

CHAPTER 2 —

GETTING CLIENTS

Marketing

Solid clinical knowledge and skills may be enough for providing good therapy. However, it is not enough to get referrals and attract clients.

Getting clients is key to building a thriving practice. But this is where many practitioners struggle.

Many therapists feel awkward about marketing.

Marketing is simply getting the word out about who you are and what you do for people.

It's telling people what you do over and over. There are many ways of telling people — in person, in writing, through the media and by phone. You have to tell them. You can't just wait for the phone to start ringing.

Marketing benefits your community because they can access the help you provide. Marketing builds your practice as it generates referrals.

This can seem like an enormous challenge for many mental health professionals. Many of us are not comfortable with promoting ourselves or our services. We tend to like to provide our helpful services, but become shy about promoting them.

Understanding more about what marketing is and some simple, effective ways to do it can help. Shedding unhelpful limiting beliefs about ourselves, marketing and what we can do and how we should do it may also be necessary.

Developing know-how and skills will also go a long way toward becoming more comfortable with marketing our practice.

Of course, our marketing and materials must be in keeping with the dignity of our profession.

Good marketing is engaging people in a consideration of taking a step that will result in their greater good. Good marketing strategies develop when we select methods that fit well with who we are as individuals.

For example, if you like to write but do not like to speak to groups, your marketing should emphasize your writing talents. Those of you who enjoy speaking and making presentations will find this is an excellent way to get the word out.

You may think, "But I'm not a business person. How can I effectively market my practice and get clients?"

Don't lose sight of why you are a therapist. Stay connected to it. But regardless of where you are in your learning about the business side of private practice, you can learn step by step how to get clients by following the Today's Private Practice approach.

By the time you finish this book, you will:

- Know where to begin to find new clients
- Have the beginnings (at least) of a strategy to reach your goals
- Have motivation to build your practice.

The key to marketing psychology services is choosing a set of simple effective things to do, and do them consistently. The Today's Private Practice system will help you do just that.

This part of the book will cover what they don't teach you in graduate school.

Choosing a Niche Market

A niche market is a group of people with common characteristics, issues and concerns. For example, attorneys, couples dealing with infertility, parents of children with ADHD, children whose parents divorced and career women over 40 are all potential niches.

Defining your services and target groups are an important step in effective marketing. It is not enough to say you are a therapist. "Therapy" is too broad and non-specific.

As we established before, marketing is simply getting the word out about what you do. Not choosing a target market or markets is like trying to get your voice heard over the din of your whole community.

You aren't going to be heard.

If you want to effectively communicate and get the word out, you need to know to whom you want to communicate.

That's the idea behind the exercise of choosing a niche market. No one can effectively market to everyone.

Great marketing goes in depth with a specific target group. Surface attempts to get the attention of the masses does not work.

Sometimes a niche can be a clinical specialty. Specialties attract clients more than a general practice. It will also attract your ideal client — the type of client and services you most enjoy in your work. Sophisticated consumers today are more likely to seek out a specialist if they can find one.

It may take some time and reflection to identify ideal niches for your practice. It may evolve over time. Or maybe one day, your niche will jump out at you.

Richard Bolles said, "Your mission is where the world's deepest hunger and your heart's greatest gladness intersect." The same can be said for identifying your niche.

Some questions to stimulate your thinking:

- Think about your previous clients. What profession was your most enjoyable client?
- What characteristic of clients do you tend to attract?
- What similar problems do your clients seem to have?
- What type of situation have you been most effective in?
- What knowledge and skills have your accumulated? How have you utilized (or underutilized) them in your work to date?

Developing a Service Line

As you define your practice, you will want to select a niche or maybe a few niches and get to know them well. You will research their felt needs and urgent concerns. You will shape your services to meet these needs and develop effective ways of communicating to your niche.

Do some market research. What are the felt needs and issues that appear to be of urgent concern to people in the target group you plan to serve? Talk to and interview a number of people in your target market to find out. Read the newsletters they read. Attend meetings they attend.

Make a list of the kinds of services you have interest in providing and what interests and energizes you.

Examples:

- Helping ADHD executives increase productivity
- Assisting struggling college students to achieve better grades
- Helping singles to have greater success in dating relationships.

The basic idea is to match the felt needs of your market with solutions that you can offer, based on what services command your interest and is within your capability. You may need to receive some training if a service is not within your current skill set.

By zeroing in on a specific niche and line of services, you will develop a competitive advantage over other providers in your area, due to your specialization. You will eventually develop a reputation for the service that will attract referrals to you.

Speaking of competition, there are advantages to having services in our line that are not covered by managed care. Although many people will opt to pay out of pocket for customized, quality services, others may not. Examples of services that are not covered by managed care include child-custody evaluations and other court-related services, psycho-educational evaluations, business consulting and coaching business owners or executives.

Other examples of specific services include resiliency training, co-parenting counseling for divorcing parents, divorce recovery groups, marriage enrichment retreats, career counseling for professionals in transition, court-ordered psychological evaluations, forensic consulting in personal injury cases, or a 10-week group for business professionals with ADHD.

Again, more traditional services, such as psychotherapy for anxiety or depression, are fine as well. There are effective ways to market these services and gather private-pay referrals. I have a steady stream of referrals based on my reputation for cognitive therapy of anxiety and depression. If this applies to you, keep it as a part of the mix.

Remember:

Niche + Problem + Format = Service

It also helps to package your services into a format that makes it easy to communicate to your target group. More on this later.

Multiple Streams of Referrals

The ultimate goal of marketing a psycholotherapy practice is to have multiple streams of referrals coming in to your office.

Clients will come to you by way of gatekeepers or referral sources, word of mouth and by getting the word out to your niche market.

Once you understand your niche market, you are in a better position to find potential clients. Circulating where your candidates come together will present opportunities to get the word out effectively.

Where do people in your target market hang out? Put yourself in front of them. Speak at their organization. Network at their meetings. Write articles for their publications. Put out a newsletter or e-zine (also called an e-newsletter).

For example, Toastmasters is an organization that helps people learn how to be a better public speaker. Anxiety is commonly a barrier for some of these individuals. In fact, people often come to Toastmasters to help themselves to become more comfortable with speaking. A practitioner could attend meetings regularly and network, or present helpful information in a talk.

Or, you can publish an article in a publication that people in your niche market reads.

It is also important to focus on the professionals who have members of your target group passing through their offices. These professionals are often in a position to make a referral for services that you may provide.

Examples include medical doctors of various specialties and PCPs, attorneys, teachers, principals, school counselors and psychologists, clergy, human resource department professionals, social workers and other mental health professionals.

Travel agents may know of people who are afraid to fly. Dentists have contact with people too fearful to keep appointments.

When you have a specialty niche, colleagues and other mental health professionals can be an excellent source of referrals, once you effectively get the word out.

Your own current and past clients are an excellent source of referrals, when they are primed to do so. Satisfied clients are a great marketing vehicle. What do you do to tactfully encourage referrals from your clients?

Who have been your best sources of referrals in the past? How can you multiply this and find several more like them?

What additional referral source relationships could you develop?

Constantly look for opportunities to develop relationships with referral sources.

For example, a client who was also being treated medically by a psychiatrist recently came into my practice. A routine phone conversation to coordinate on treatment led to me talking about my services. I received three referrals from this psychiatrist in the following month.

How can you develop connections with referral sources?

Keep in mind that a brief encounter with a referral source will not likely result in a stream of referrals. Usually, a relationship must be built. People refer to professionals they know, like and trust.

So, look at getting referral streams as relationship building — something therapists do routinely. Set up lunch or coffee meetings, or send them your newsletter and occasional items of interest, such as an article you think they may be interested in reading. Over time, they may become a valuable source of referrals.

The Marketing Cycle

The key to getting clients and referrals for clients is giving people the opportunity to know, like and trust you. This happens more readily when you have a process in place. This process is called The Marketing Cycle.

There are four stages to The Marketing Cycle:

1. Filling the reservoir of contacts
2. Following up
3. Getting presentations
4. Adding clients/gathering referrals

1. Filling the Reservoir

We fill our reservoir of contacts (prospective clients or referral sources) by meeting people through the course of our business, such as telephone contact with clients' PCP or previous therapist, or through outreach strategies like networking or speaking.

Your goal is to keep adding to the reservoir regularly.

Other ways we can fill the reservoir include:

- Networking
- Referral building
- Public speaking
- Writing — for magazines and newsletters
- Promotional events
- Advertising
- Publicity (being interviewed in the newspaper or a magazine)
- Internet marketing

2. Following Up

It's important to follow up with people you meet who seem interested in your services.

Some people will be ready to become a client or referral source immediately, but many will need time and additional contact.

Remember, they need to know, like and trust you.

So, see if you can set up a time to have a conversation. In this conversation, you will find out more about his/her needs, tell him/her more about what you do and see if there is a match. This conversation is also referred to as a presentation of your services.

Some people will not be ready for this. Others will not be ready to become a client or send you referrals regularly. So, you want a system in place by which you can follow up with contacts, and remind them of your services on an ongoing basis.

People often need to hear about you several times before they are ready.

Following up can be done through a periodic newsletter, which helps keep your name in front of people so they don't forget you, or through further conversations over lunch, coffee or the telephone.

Following up can also happen through sending out information pieces about your services through brochures and announcements.

3. Getting Presentations

Actual presentations can be formal or informal, and can happen in person, by telephone or by mail or email.

For example, you may set up a lunch with a professional who sees people in your target market. During lunch, you demonstrate an interest in his/her business, and ask him/her more about it and the types of clients who are ideal for him/her. The professional reciprocates and asks you about your practice.

You give a brief overview of your services (presentation) and who your target group is (the profile of your ideal client).

When talking about your services, be clear about the value you offer. Speak to the benefits of your services that your clients receive.

Be sure to follow up. If things go well, you will want to build a relationship over time.

So, regularly remind them that you are out there, and thank them for referrals.

4. Adding Clients

Sometimes making a presentation will result in a person becoming a client or making a referral to you. If not, you may need to make another presentation or continue following up with them as long as it seems worthwhile.

I have had situations in which a person heard me speak at his/her organization and became a client a year later.

What the marketing cycle looks like for your practice will depend on the type of services you provide and what is natural for you.

What needs the most work at this point in your practice — filling the reservoir, following up, getting presentations or adding clients?

Are you stuck in any of these areas? If so, make this the focus of your efforts for the next few weeks.

Marketing and Who You Are

Don't feel discouraged if marketing your practice seems daunting at first. There are many ways of getting the word out, some of them more naturally suited to who you are and some not. You will want to identify strategies that fit well with who you are.

Each of us is unique and will use a different approach.

At the same time, some of us may need to get over our blocks about marketing. Irrational beliefs will impede your progress.

One of my coaching clients, a bright and talented psychologist, was struggling to move forward in starting his private practice. He was experiencing fear and reluctance. As we explored the cause for this, we uncovered the irrational belief that he had, which was: "I am not good enough. I am not talented enough as a therapist." Knowing him, this was not true. Together we were able to work on this interference and soon he was taking the steps he needed to effectively build his practice.

At the root of our fears are doubts and negative beliefs about ourselves and the world. These thoughts impede you from operating outside of your comfort zone. They can act to paralyze you. Eliminating any irrational fears you have that weaken your resolve and ability to act is an important step.

See if any of these negative beliefs sound familiar:

- "I'm not good enough."
- "It will never work."
- "That's only true for others, not for me."
- "I can't change"
- "I can't be successful."

Once negative beliefs are identified and dealt with, you will want to find a set of marketing strategies that fits well with who you are.

There are many good strategies for marketing a private practice, including direct contact, networking, public speaking, writing, promotional events and advertising.

The suitability of a particular strategy can depend on the situation. Direct contact with potential clients may be an inappropriate strategy for a psychotherapy service. Therefore, it may be good to rely more on networking and referral building. However, it can be a good strategy to use for connecting with referral sources.

The selection of strategies also depends on who you are and your preferences, strengths and abilities. For example, a poor public speaker would do well to focus more on writing and publicity instead.

To what are you naturally drawn and what will you actually do? For example, if you are outgoing and enjoy talking to people, choose actions that will get you to networking events. If you choose activities you like or are willing to try, you are more likely to do them.

Utilizing effective strategies may involve getting out of your comfort zone and learning some new skills. This was definitely true for me. I was not highly comfortable or skilled at networking several years ago, but it has become a growth area for me that has helped build my practice significantly.

Get Out of the Office

One mistake I see many practitioners make at the start of their private practice is that they select only passive marketing strategies in finding clients and referral sources. They wait for people to come to them, rather than take a more active approach to go out and meet people.

Marketing strategies can be active or passive. Sometimes our fears of not knowing what to say, appearing foolish or being rejected cause us to gravitate towards passive approaches.

Passive marketing strategies include sending out letters, brochures and newsletters, writing articles and advertising.

Active marketing strategies include attending networking venues and events, calling contacts and leads, meeting people over coffee or lunch and giving presentations to organizations.

Guess which strategies are more effective? While passive marketing strategies have an important place in our practice-building efforts, the active strategies are much more effective.

So, get out of the office!

Developing a Plan

Where do clients come from? They come from having a set of simple, effective marketing strategies, and marketing consistently.

In my coaching work with other therapists, we often work together on tailoring a marketing plan specific to their own situation.

An interesting phenomenon happens when they get serious and focused on consistent marketing; they get results in unexpected ways. Prospects they talked to three months ago suddenly call, saying they are interested in working with them. Someone they meet seems like a great prospect. They get a referral from someone they don't even remember.

But, these are not accidents. They are the results of effort put into marketing. They are the result of meeting people and developing skills in articulating services. Although sometimes the results seem accidental, they are connected to consistent, planned marketing efforts.

A marketing plan consists of a set of actions that gets you clients, combined with the tools, information and skills you need to help you fill your reservoir of contacts, follow up and get presentations.

These actions include things like:

- Sending a mailing
- Meeting people in your target group
- Going to a networking event
- Contacting groups or organizations about speaking
- Writing an article
- Attending a professional meeting
- Having lunch with a referral source
- Contacting potential referral partners
- Sending an item of interest to a colleague
- Making follow-up calls
- Distributing fliers to organizations
- Doing something to get your name in print

Marketing tools, information and skills are the success ingredients that facilitate and increase the effectiveness of your actions.

These are things like:

- A description of your services
- A succinct, well-articulated statement of who you are and what you do
- Business cards
- A list of appropriate networking venues
- Networking skills
- A list of possible speaking venues
- Information pieces such as brochures
- A contact management system, preferably on computer
- A newsletter
- Target market research
- A presentation script or talking points
- Biography sheet
- Web site
- Personal mailing list
- Speaking skills

What are the missing ingredients for your marketing efforts? What tools, information or skills do you need to develop to move you forward?

With a good plan and the right tools you are better positioned to see success in getting clients. The magic formula is selecting a set of simple, effective things to do and doing them consistently.

You make the best selections when you take into account who you are. So...

- Know and use your natural talents.
- Find your paths of least resistance and focus on these.
- Expect some fear and awkwardness at first — it's natural.

For more information about marketing strategies, I recommend the following books:

1) "Get Clients Now" by C. J. Hayden
2) "Power Networking" by Donna Fisher and Sandy Vilas

The Today's Private Practice web site has a wealth of useful resources, tips and techniques. See www.TodaysPrivatePractice.com.

12 Marketing Ideas to Build Your Practice That You Can Implement Right Away

1. Create brochures for your general practice and for each specialty or niche service.

2. Develop or polish your networking skills and network with strategic professionals (referral sources) and/or members of your niche market.

3. Develop a seminar or workshop related to your niche service.

4. Have a monthly or quarterly newsletter and send it to referral sources, clients and past clients and other people you have met through networking.

5. Host an open house and send out invitations to get the attention of referral sources and develop relationships.

6. Use a press release when you have a special event or noteworthy happening to get exposure in the community or niche.

7. Do a presentation at a convention, local organization meeting or even a "lunch-and-learn" talk at a local business.

8. Offer a training program or continuing education course for your colleagues or even your referral sources.

9. Offer a health screening to reach into your community or niche.

10. Write articles for publications as well as for distributing to clients, referral sources and others.

11. Give psychology away by volunteering some time in meeting community needs.

12. Your clients can be one of your best referral sources, so inform them and keep them aware of your services through brochures and articles in your waiting room and sending them your newsletter.

CHAPTER 3 —

THE EIGHT STEPS

To organize your efforts, you may find the following eight-step process useful.

1. Find a Niche

To niche or not to niche? There are many advantages to focusing your practice on a niche or set of niches, as described previously.

Specialties attract more clients than a general practice.

So, how do you decide on a niche?

To start with, look for the convergence of three factors:

1) What do you love to do? What type of clients, services or work do you thrive on the most? What are you passionate about?

2) What you are best at? Where do your talents lie? What do you have the potential to become the best at in your locale or region? What are your favorite skills?

3) What is lucrative? Will people pay for this service? Is there potential to have well-paying clients for this?

When you find a niche service that taps into these three factors, you have a potentially good niche.

Does that stimulate any ideas?

Ideally, you will find an underserved area that will continue to grow. For example, in my area, there are a shortage of child psychiatrists and play therapists.

Do some market research. Look in the media. What are the urgent concerns and felt needs that people have?

Your personal and professional experiences may give you some good ideas.

Colleagues may also be a good source of ideas. What are they talking about in the way of innovative psychological services?

To see what other professionals on the entrepreneurial side are doing, see the monthly newsletter Psychotherapy Finances (visit www.PsyFin.com for more information). Each issue contains at least one article about what practioners are successfully developing as niches.

(Appendix I contains a working list of possible niche markets.)

2. Discover the Niche Markets' Problems

What are the felt needs, which are not always the same as real needs, of the niche group?

How can you find out? Do some market research. Review literature on this target group. What are articles in relevant publications discussing? Read publications that people in this niche market read.

One of the best ways to do this research is to sit down over lunch with an individual in your niche market and interview him/her. While you are at it, you can also test market some of the ideas you have for services and programs you might offer to see what kind of reaction you get.

Another way might be to conduct a poll, forum or focus group. Survey the needs of your niche.

Know your target market.

(Appendix 2 is a working list of possible felt needs in various niche markets.)

3. Develop Solutions

How can you help meet the felt needs and address the urgent concerns of your niche market?

Decide on a service or set of services you can offer that will help the niche market with its challenges in an effective way.

To get ideas for this service, research the literature on what may be an effective treatment. Obtain training and supervision as needed. Are there any programs or approaches that you can adapt?

Example:

Niche Market: Heart surgery patients, post-surgery.

Problem: Compliance with post-surgery health recommendations, such as medication regimen, diet and exercise programs.

Solution: A behavioral health component to the aftercare program to help with cardiac care compliance. Some therapists are doing this with good results and profits.

Think in terms of a range of services for the niche market: workshops, groups, psychotherapy, consultation and coaching.

4. Design Packaging

Packaging is important.

After you have identified a solution for your niche market's felt needs, I suggest you develop it into a step-by-step program.

Clients understand products easier than services, which are less tangible.

An example of a mental health package or product is a stress-management program with:

- A set of curriculum
- A workbook
- A fixed price

Have a process that you deliver. Let your prospective clients know you have as plan and a process to help them.

This gives you more credibility and the potential client hope that it will be beneficial.

The process description answers the questions about how you help people and what you would do with them in therapy.

Delineate the steps of your process in a way that leads a person to say, "I want that."

There are several other advantages to this. One is the way this will crystallize your thinking. You will also become much more articulate in describing the features and benefits of your services.

Now you have a marketable service to add to your service line.

For example, years ago, I identified divorced parents embroiled in high conflict over their co-parenting issues as a niche market. This, as we know, has harmful affects on the children and causes stress for the parents. And it's a common problem.

My solution was to do targeted counseling with these parents on co-parenting more collaboratively.

I packaged this into a six- to 12-session program I called, "Cooperative Co-parenting for Divorcing Parents." I outlined a five-step program and wrote a booklet describing the steps. This became a good marketing tool as well as an aid for my clients. (Niche + Problem + Program = Service)

- Pick a niche market
- Identify a specific problem that the niche market experiences
- Develop a program to deliver your solution

5. Develop a Marketing Plan

Consumers do not know you or what you do unless you communicate that to them. Develop a plan to let people know what you do, how you can help them and how they can contact you.

For each service in your repertoire, write a marketing plan.

How will you fill your reservoir of contacts and attract people to your practice?

To whom will you market this service? What strategies will you use? What tools do you need to develop?

For example, for my Cooperative Co-parenting program, I realized that the target group for marketing this service was often not the embattled parents or the children, but the family court judges who would mandate the service and the divorce attorneys who see the struggling parents in their offices.

I developed a brochure as well as the booklet mentioned previously, and handed them out to many judges and attorneys with whom I networked.

A basic marketing plan will outline each service in your service line, each services' target market and several strategies to promote your service to the target group.

How will you establish yourself as an expert in this area? Develop, disseminate and repeat your message to each target market.

How will you create opportunities to interact with your referral sources and prospective clients?

6. Implement Marketing

This is sometimes more challenging than it sounds.

Besides the challenge of initial inertia, there is the challenge of getting good and comfortable with articulating your services in a way that will connect with your target market.

I find that many mental health professionals are not great at articulating their services in laymen's terms.

So, consider how you can develop your skills in doing this.

One helpful exercise would be to write out a 30-second commercial or description about the service and get feedback on it. Once you have a good one, practice it until it's natural.

Marketing skills and execution get better with time, experience and practice.

To get the word out about you, become a good communicator so people can understand the impact that your services can offer. A business coach can be very beneficial with this step as well as the other seven.

Your task is to develop a referral engine.

Build a self-generating engine that keeps going easily and yields a steady flow of referrals.

You might do this by some or all of the following:

- Schedule a networking lunch with different referral sources each month.
- Give free talks to organizations.
- Send out a mailing every month or every quarter to your mailing list of past clients, referral sources and others.
- Get out of the office and meet people. Expand your mailing list by 10 names each month.

To work out a plan for marketing, you will need to set aside some time on a weekly basis. To be successful, you will have to make marketing a priority and consistently engage in the most strategic activities.

7. Create a Follow-Up System

For those who do not initially accept your services, have a follow-up system in place.

The goal of marketing is to get prospective clients or referral sources to know, like and trust you. This usually takes multiple exposures to you over time.

A follow-up system makes sure you keep in contact with valuable referral sources and prospects and exposes them to you over and over.

Examples of elements in a follow-up system include a periodic newsletter, a database of contacts, periodic coffee or lunch appointments with referral sources and appearances at venues where these people circulate.

In addition, I regularly mail a brochure about each of my services to the target groups of each service.

You will, in time, accumulate a valuable mailing or e-mailing list and referral sources. I find each time I mail out the periodic newsletter or brochures, my phone starts ringing in the coming weeks with referrals as people are reminded of my services.

8. Keep it Going and Growing

Some suggestions to keep things going and growing:

- Maintain balance in your life and good self-care.
- Be persistent and persevere.
- Find support in friends, colleagues and referral partners.
- Develop and maintain good business systems. Automate things as much as possible. Invest in a good computer, software and telephone system.
- Maintain quality services.
- Provide excellent customer service.

The TodaysPrivatePractice.com members resource area has many helpful and practical articles and resources for each of the eight steps. It's there to support you.

CHAPTER 4 —

STREAMS OF PSYCHOTHERAPY INCOME

Mental health professionals have a wealth of valuable, even crucial, information and expertise in which many people are in need.

One-on-one therapy is only one way we can deliver this expertise and help.

In this section, I will discuss a number of possible ways therapists can create revenue streams while sharing their talents, expertise and skills with people in need.

Some of these ways are traditional and common, but others are rather innovative ways therapists are beginning to put their abilities to good use. In doing so, they are creating revenue streams.

Traditional Services

Although this book suggests its time for therapists to think out of the box and develop new services that creatively meet the felt needs of niche markets, there is a place for the traditional therapeutic services.

These include psychotherapy for the DSM diagnoses, psychological testing and evaluation, marriage and family therapy and behavioral health care.

And, yes, people will forgo managed-care reimbursement and pay out of pocket for services that are of higher value because they are higher quality, offer real privacy and are truly customized for the individual needs.

Much of what is encouraged in this book applies to the marketing of traditional services. This is where niche marketing can be especially valuable.

One of the frustrations I hear from mental health care service consumers is that they can't find a specialized therapist in their managed-care insurance network.

It's as if managed care's philosophy is, "We'll help you obtain access to psychotherapy, but we don't care whether the therapist we connect you with is a specialist. A generalist is fine."

Set yourself apart and demonstrate your true value in the marketplace through specialization. Many people in the market for therapy value specialization.

Years ago I developed a specialization in the area of assessing and treating Attention Deficit Hyperactivity Disorder. This niche has been a consistent stream of referrals ever since.

I thoroughly researched the area, saw many clients with ADHD, became published in professional books and journals, created booklets and materials for my clients, served on the board of a local CHADD organization and presented seminars and workshops.

More recently, I created a very simple web site that presents numerous resources for individuals affected by ADHD (www.ManageADD.com). The web site offers a wealth of information and resources, including articles, an e-book, book recommendations and recommended web site links, as well as highlights my practice and services in this niche.

Getting Published

A book is a powerful way to affect lives. It is also a good way to establish credibility, highlight your practice and services and position yourself in your niche.

And, it's easier than you think if you self-publish. It has become very affordable to do so, and it puts you in charge of the content, price and reprints.

It can actually be more profitable, too. You keep every dollar above your costs. If you went through a major publisher who sells a few thousand books, you would only receive the author's fee. You can make as much selling a few hundred copies of a self-published book yourself.

If your book is successful, you may even attract a large publisher to take over your book.

Writing a book opens doors to speaking engagements, media opportunities and a reputation in your niche market.

It also helps you to crystallize your thinking and enhances your effectiveness as a practitioner; it's a great exercise in that sense. You will learn a lot both in breadth and depth.

Take the opportunity now to brainstorm ideas for a book that's inside you.

It doesn't have to be long. One hundred pages is plenty.

Teaching

Teaching courses part-time at a local college or university can be an attractive stream of income.

I have been teaching as adjunct faculty in the Doctor of Psychology (Psy.D.) program at Widener University outside Philadelphia for several years and find it both rewarding and enjoyable.

Think about areas of special interest on which you could teach a course. Courses that adjunct faculty teach can be core curriculum in a graduate program, an undergraduate course or an elective.

I find that part-time professors who are practioners have a lot to offer because they are immersed in what they teach. Students seem to appreciate this as well.

Remaining connected with academia can be very enjoyable and rewarding.

I am a firm believer that having a good mix in your work can help battle against burnout. Variety keeps you stimulated, challenged and interested in your work.

One of the great things about a profession in mental health is that there is such a variety available to us in our work. Teaching can be a good part of this mix.

E-books

E-books are another medium in which you can package and share specialized information.

And e-book is a written piece of information that is distributed via the internet electronically. It is offered free or for a cost (typically $10 to $30) on a web site.

You can also submit an e-book to web sites that list hundreds of e-books to make them available to the public.

Tens of thousands of e-books are downloaded each year, and are changing lives for the better.

Perhaps you can make yours one of them.

Do you have a solution to a specific problem or can you research the answers?

The best e-books share answers to a specific problem.

E-book topics I have heard of recently include: how to write a eulogy, how to cope with a hysterectomy and the topic of recovering from fibromyalgia.

For example, see www.EulogyHelpDesk.com. The e-book "A Eulogy to Remember" is offered to individuals needing immediate help with this task.

Or visit www.HappyHysterectomy.com, where "The Worried Woman's Guide to a Happy Hysterectomy" e-book can be obtained.

These are e-books written by non-mental health professionals. Imagine what information psychotherapists can offer in this just-in-time format.

E-books cost very little to produce and nothing to distribute. You can attach the file for an e-book to an email or make it downloadable from a web site.

A great e-book is not long. Many of the best are 10 to 35 pages long.

E-books offer short answers to problems readers want to solve, and are available to people quickly.

Good e-books are specific and do not contain general information. The key to marketability is communicating your precise answer to a specific problem.

As you prepare to write an e-book, read other good ones and see what makes them valuable.

Email me at info@TodaysPrivatePractice.com, and I will send you an example of an e-book I wrote titled, "Fitness for the Mind: Dealing With the Negative Beliefs that Hold You Back."

E-courses

E-courses are similar to e-books, but they may be lengthier and delivered to readers one segment at a time. As the name implies, these can be formatted as guided self-study programs.

E-courses allow for the content to be integrated over a specific period of time. Each lesson can be a simple article or more in-depth with guided self-study. Write between five and 10 lessons, and you have a good e-course.

Written by a professional, a good e-course can bridge the gap between a reader learning new information and the reader applying that information to his/her life and making a behavioral change.

Personal Coaching

In sports, coaching is important to help an athlete develop a winning strategy, develop skills and execute the plan. The coach knows how the athlete can progress and move forward. He/she urges the athlete to set high goals and provides motivation, support, focus and encouragement.

Over the past 10 years, the field of professional coaching in personal development and business arenas has grown tremendously.

What is coaching? Personal coaching is a one-on-one professional relationship in which a client is assisted in achieving a personal, business or career goal.

What is the difference between coaching and therapy? Although coaches sometimes assist people with challenges and problems of various kinds, they do not try to help people overcome problems related to diagnosable conditions as found in the DSM. Rather, coaches assist well-functioning people to attain greater levels of achievement and satisfaction in their personal lives, businesses or careers.

While therapy is remedial and restorative, coaching is developmental and growth-oriented.

Therapy heals mental and emotional infirmities, while coaching helps healthy individuals achieve more or reach important goals.

Personal coaches work with clients on a wide range of issues, such as coping with a problem or crisis, focusing their efforts on achievement, making career transitions, living more fulfilled lives, achieving life goals and building better relationships.

Other coaches assist people with business development or managerial or leadership development. These coaches are called business coaches or executive coaches.

While coaching is not always based on psychology, it often is. And many of the skills a coach uses are the skills in which therapists are trained. So, there is considerable overlap between coaching and therapy.

This is why many psychologists, counselors and therapists have found coaching attractive and transitioned into coaching either entirely or as a part of their practice mix. I am one of them.

In many ways, therapists have an ideal background to be coaches. But the differences between coaching and therapy are significant and important to keep in mind.

For more information on coaching, the following books and web sites are recommended:

1) "Therapist as Life Coach: Transforming Your Practice" by Patrick Williams and Deborah C. Davis (2002).

2) "Personal and Executive Coaching: The Complete Guide for Mental Health Professionals" by Jeffery Averbach, Ph.D. (2001).

3) The International Coach Federation (ICF), the guiding body for professional coaches, can be found at www.CoachFederation.org.

4) The Philadelphia Area Coaches Alliance (PACA), one of the larger local organizations of coaches, can be found at www.PhiladelphiaCoaches.org.

For additional information, visit my web site, which includes my executive, business and career coaching services, www.LeadershipConcepts.net.

Therapists can make great coaches because of their insights into human motivation and behavior, their understanding of human development and life transitions, their communication and relationship skill and their sense of professional ethics, knowledge base and experience in helping people.

Live Workshops, Retreats, Trainings

Presenting live events such as seminars, workshops, retreats and training programs can be a very lucrative stream of income.

And, it can be a powerful way to affect peoples' lives.

The group setting allows learners to engage with your material and benefit from the collective knowledge and experience of the group.

Live programs can also be an introduction to your other services. Brief programs, such as a "lunch and learn," can be delivered for free as a solid marketing vehicle for your practice.

As a therapist, if you have developed and packaged your message into a program as recommended earlier, you have the makings of a great seminar or workshop.

Why not kill two birds with one stone?

Promoting a workshop or retreat is promoting your practice at the same time — and may be psychologically easier to do.

Consider adding a post-training element to your program. It could be a follow-up mini-workshop, a series of workshops or one-on-one work.

You can leverage the energy of a live event in many ways for additional revenue streams. And, it is likely that some participants will choose to work with you after the event is over.

You will want to casually present your other offerings at the event. You may make it easier for them by having a sign-up sheet.

Visit www.AdaptivLearning.com to learn more about Adaptiv Learning Systems, which develops, markets and delivers training programs that teach people to become more resilient in the midst of life's challenges. Their resiliency training programs are based on the work of well-known University of Pennsylvania professor of psychology Dr. Martin Seligman, past President of the American Psychological Association.

Dr. Seligman's recent book, Authentic Happiness, and the web site www.AuthenticHappiness.org are other examples of the type of services and products in the personal growth/skills-building genre that mental health professionals can offer.

See also www.DifficultChild.com for the offerings of Howard Glasser, M.A., as an example. His web site highlights his Nurtured Heart Approach program of parenting behaviorally challenged children, as well as his book, workshops, training, therapy and coaching material.

Teleseminars

A teleseminar (also called a teleclass) is a seminar held over the telephone, like a conference call.

The advantage of a teleseminar is the convenience. No one has to commute and the consumers dial to a bridge line at the specified time. No physical accommodations need be arranged; you only need to rent a telephone bridgeline.

Teleseminars can include people from all over the country, even internationally, at the same time.

Classes are typically 60 minutes long, but can vary. Often teleseminars are offered in a multi-class series.

Teleseminars are another way to offer your packaged content and introduce people to your services. Teleseminars can be offered for free to attract prospective clients and let them sample your services.

See www.TeleClass.com for examples of what various professionals are offering. Or, do a search on Google for teleseminars or teleclasses. There are hundreds to browse and attend.

To get a better feel for how to conduct a teleseminar, attend several yourself (you can attend offerings free as a member of TodaysPrivatePractice.com).

What are some topics on which you could host a one-hour teleseminar?

Consulting

The goal of this book is to help mental health practitioners build thriving managed-care free private practices.

One of the themes I hope I have conveyed is that psychology is not just for DSM diagnoses.

While we have discussed ways to market traditional services, diversification is important, as it increases the chances we can generate sufficient income to operate outside of managed care.

Multiple streams of psychotherapy income can be developed in one's practice.

When I decided to build a manage-care free practice, I gave considerable thought to how I could provide private-pay services. I explored how I could use my skills in ways that people would readily pay.

Many psychologists and other mental health professionals are successful in consulting in the workplace for the benefit of employees and employers. Business consulting can be a very lucrative income stream.

Like many practitioners, I found my skills could be applied in the business arena. Today, through a business I started called Leadership Concepts (www.LeadershipConcepts.net), I offer services in the areas of business consulting, executive, business and career coaching and seminars and workshops for businesses. This has proven to be a solid and growing income stream for me, and it is work I really enjoy.

Other ways to diversify into consulting include behavioral medicine, forensics and sports psychology.

Consulting is a very broad and diverse area, so I won't scrape the surface of the possibilities here. But perhaps I can give you good directions for exploration.

If this area is new for you, you will be surprised to find out the many valuable ways our psychology and mental health expertise can be of benefit to people in the workplace.

Our background makes us capable of assisting businesses with many different barriers to productivity, including:

- A company with a morale problem
- A department not functioning well as a team
- A conflict between key individuals in a business
- A leader with underdeveloped interpersonal skills
- A crisis or setback that has traumatized workers
- A downsizing

To familiarize yourself with this terrain, I suggest you do a Google search using the keywords "business," "consulting" and "psychologist" and browse the web sites that come up.

A good book on business consulting is "Flawless Consulting: A Guide to Getting Your Expertise Used" by Peter Block.

For a psychology-based approach to business consulting, see "Psychological Consulting to Management" by Lester Tobias (1990) and "Executive Coaching" by Richard Kilburg (2000).

Forensic Consulting

Another specific type of consulting is worth considering separately.

Forensic consulting has to do with psychological or mental health service specifically related to the court system.

Often times, a court has to deal with issues that impinge on mental health issues.

Some of these include:

Criminal cases

- Competency to stand trial
- Mental status at time of offense
- Mitigating factors in offenses
- Risk assessments, violence

Civil cases

- Emotional damages in personal injuries
- Assessments for malingering

Family cases and other

- Child custody evaluations
- Court-ordered psychological evaluations

In addition, attorneys often need help sorting out the issues when questions of a psychological nature occur in their cases. They retain psychologists and other experts to review files and help them prepare for depositions or cross-examination of experts.

Psychologists and other professionals can inform the court on issues, perform assessments and testify as experts.

Consultants in this area testifying as experts typically receive $1,000 to $2,000 for their testimony.

I find that this niche is an attractive one for several reasons:

- It is completely managed-care free
- It is interesting work
- It makes good use of our background
- It is lucrative
- It is a specialized area that many professionals find intimidating, which means less competition.

If you find this an interesting prospect as a part of your practice, then I encourage you to begin taking some training workshops to familiarize yourself with the arena, and then proceed to retool yourself so that you can ethically operate as a forensic consultant.

I recommend the workshops and materials available through the American Academy of Forensic Psychology (www.ABFP.com).

Web sites

Revenue streams can be active or passive. Therapy sessions, therapy groups, workshops and consulting services are all active forms of revenue streams. You exchange your time and skills for a fee.

Passive revenue is revenue from streams that do not involve service delivery, but once set up, occur automatically 24/7. A common form of passive revenue is income from products sold on a web site.

Can you see the advantages of passive revenue? Can therapists develop passive revenue streams? You bet!

Therapists can productize their most useful expertise and offer information products to benefit others.

Some of these we already looked at, like books, e-books and e-courses. These can all be offered on a web site for web seekers to obtain and utilize to fill their needs.

There are other possibilities as well, such as licensing programs.

As an example of a passive revenue web site effectively offering information products to a specific niche, see www.TeachMe-Teamwork.com.

Passive income streams utilizing the internet via web sites are a burgeoning area for many service professionals, but few mental health professionals are taking advantage of the potential so far.

This will be changing soon.

Active income streams can also be marketed on the internet.

Web sites can also be effectively used as a marketing tool for your fee-for-service practice. More and more therapists are putting up web sites and for good reasons.

A web site is your practice brochure, available any time, day or night, to seekers on the internet. People you meet, people who hear you give a presentation and people referred to you by another professional, can be directed to view your web site, find out more about you and, hopefully, be stimulated to contact you.

A simple, attractive, intriguing postcard sent to a mailing list can direct your niche market to your web site. Or, your yellow page ad in the phone book can include your web address.

A web site is much more than a brochure. It is also a potentially powerful marketing vehicle, when combined with internet marketing strategies.

If you decide to have a web site for your practice, or for a particular niche service, make it full of resources (articles and free information) that will attract people to it and make them want to spread the word.

Although beyond the scope of this book, internet marketing strategies can be developed to drive people to your web site.

Increasingly, people are beginning their search for products and services on the internet. The yellow pages are not the first choice for many.

Are you effectively represented on the Internet?

Licensing Programs

After you have developed effective structured programs for your niches, you can license the use of these programs to other professionals.

Other therapists have been doing this for years. Psychologist Dr. Daniel Dana, a conflict resolution specialist, certifies mediators and licenses his program at www.MediationWorks.com.

Another example can be found at www.DifficultChild.com, as we mentioned previously. Howard Glasser, M.A. offers a parenting approach and program, as well as other materials, for ADHD children. His program involves a book, a training program for parents and a training and certification program for therapists.

His program is called "Transforming the Difficult Child: The Nurtured Heart Approach." One of my coaching clients is certified in this program and speaks highly of it.

Howard Glasser's web site actually models several streams of income, including a book, workshops, training other professionals, licensing or certification and internet marketing for all the above including his practice.

These "programs in a box" are typically complete turnkey therapy, counseling or consulting programs that therapists can purchase. They are usually complete, including the structured program itself, instructor materials, workbooks and also include marketing pieces you can use to generate business.

For those of you who want to do niche marketing but prefer not to do the creating part, you may want to find out whether someone has developed a program you can utilize to serve your niche.

Someone may have done the work for you.

If you can find a program suitable for your niche market, you could be a few days away from having a marketable service in your repertoire.

When developing or choosing a licensed program, there should be:

- A limited number of licenses, so that licensees will not be competing with each other.
- A clear and thorough facilitator's manual.

Training Other Professionals

When you have developed an effective program, you can leverage it by training others in your approach and methods.

Innovators in therapy have been training others for years. If you develop a specialization, program or niche service in a growing area, you may find many other therapists would like to learn from you.

Dr. Daniel Dana, the conflict resolution and mediation specialist mentioned earlier is an example (see www.MediationWorks.com). He made his reputation consulting for businesses and training managers in conflict resolution, and then began training other professionals in his program. He offers a certification program.

Sometimes the innovation is mainly in how a service is packaged.

You can train other professionals via live workshops, self-study program packages and teleseminars.

Chapter 5 —

Transitioning

The Key Concepts

There are several key concepts I invite you to consider.

It is possible to break free of managed care and thrive in private practice.

You can design and create a great practice and make a good living in your profession.

Psychology is not just for people with DSM diagnoses.

Diversification by developing a number of streams of psychology income increases the chances you can generate sustainable income and can be rewarding in other ways, too.

Niche marketing is an important strategy in today's private practice. Niche + Problem + Program = Service

Develop a service line based on for what people feel a need, what you love to do and for what people will be willing to pay.

Develop multiple streams of referrals for each service through a set of simple, effective, low-cost marketing strategies that suit your personality and target market.

Practitioners in today's private practice benefit from becoming more business-minded and entrepreneurial, more skilled in communicating their services to their niche market and getting out of the office more.

There is no scarcity of opportunity to make an impact in people's lives through psychology. You've read about a variety of ways to create revenue streams for yourself.

You've just read about several ways to generate streams of psychology income. Additional suggestions are covered in hands-on fashion at the Today's Private Practice web site (www.TodaysPrivatePractice.com).

As a mental health professional, you understand the nature of transitions. There are often barriers and sticking points along the way.

There may be limiting beliefs about what you can do to shed.

There may be periods of discomfort.

What can you do to accelerate your way to your ideal practice? That's what this section of the book is about.

This section outlines a handful of things I hope will ease the transition.

As I've gone through the transition myself and helped others as well, these are the things that seem to help.

Vision

The saying goes, "If you aim at nothing, you'll hit it every time."

Having a clear vision of where you want to go with your practice will help guide your efforts and assure that you'll end up with a practice that is truly satisfying. It will also create energy for completing the tasks involved in building a practice.

Having a vision for your practice makes everything else you do much easier. Based on your vision, choices about location, marketing, networking, training and use of time are clearer.

I encourage you to begin to develop a practice vision by engaging in a simple exercise.

In writing, describe your ideal practice in detail. Consider:

- What your days and hours of work will be
- What your clients will be like
- What you do with your clients
- How much you will be paid for your services
- How you get clients and referrals
- What revenue streams you have
- What your office environment is like
- What level of satisfaction you and your clients have
- How your practice orients around your strengths and talents, who you are, and your values

I hope that your vision speaks to you, pulling you forward to make many positive changes in your practice and your life.

Making your vision a reality will require commitment, work, follow-through and the investment of time and money.

The Business of Private Practice

Along the way of developing a thriving private practice, you will need to understand how to run a business.

One thing that is key to successful private practice is developing some proficiencies in the business of psychotherapy as well as in the craft. See yourself as a business owner.

But you don't have to be a business person to get started and be successful in private practice.

If you work at it, you can learn the basics step-by-step of how to run a business, as thousands of psychology and other professionals starting businesses do each year.

Regardless of where you are in the learning process, you can start now by learning on the job following the Today's Private Practice approach.

And, as much as you learn the business of private practice, stay connected to the spirit of why you are in the business.

Why do you practice in mental health?

Money

Think of the figure you would like to set as your financial goal for your practice. Imagine your annual income goal.

If we take the amount of $120,000 as an example, the challenge of building a private practice to reach that number can seem daunting.

When you break down a large financial goal into chunks it becomes more readily achievable and your chances of success are greater.

Using the Today's Private Practice approach, it's easier to get your arms around it.

Consider this: If 20 people pay you $120 per session for 50 weeks, that's $120,000 over the course of a year.

Do you see how the formula works? Twenty people at $110 per session for 50 weeks equals $110,000. Twenty people at $150 per session equals $150,000, and so on.

But, what if you had additional streams of income in your service line?

It could be from testing, groups, consulting, workshops, teaching and e-books.

You could make $6,000 per year teaching a couple courses at a university.

If you sell 20 copies a month of a $29 e-book, you will gross $6,960 in one year.

Or you might sell licenses to your trademark programs, copies of a book you write or collect fees for workshops or retreats.

One way you could achieve your goal is as a practice made up of the following components:

1. Psychotherapy 10 clients per week ($120 a session) $60,000

2. Teaching two courses per year at $3,000 each $6,000

3. Psychological testing at $2,500 per evaluation
(one per month) $30,000

4. Business consulting 100 hours at $200 per hour $20,000

Total gross income annually $116,000

OR

1. Psychotherapy 10 clients per week ($120 a session) $60,000

2. Personal coaching 10 clients at $300 per month.........$ 30,000

3. Psychological testing, $2,500 per month $30,000

4. Live workshops $20,000

Total gross income annually $140,000

Do these examples help you see how doable it is?

What are your financial targets? How can you break these down into revenue streams that reach your goal?

Beef Up Your Systems

By increasing and improving your systems, you can increase your capacity for work.

One of the nice things about being managed-care free is the reduction of administrative work.

However, unless you have support staff, there will still be many administrative tasks you will need to do. These can be time- and energy-consuming.

Free up time and energy and increase your capacity for work by putting good systems in place.

Systematize repetitive tasks to make them quicker and easier. Automate as much as possible.

Obtain the technology to reduce your administrative time. Get a good computer and powerful software applications specific to what you need to do.

I have found good email and contact management software are invaluable. Microsoft Outlook helps in my marketing and client management through its contact management capabilities. Also, I can easily send email to a list of people and create and distribute newsletters via email.

Good systems enable you to get more done in less time, and free you up for more leisure time.

When you run a business on your own, it pays to invest in good systems.

Therapists, Take Your Own Medicine — Work on Yourself

Work on yourself, who you want to be and the lifestyle you want for yourself and your family.

What limiting beliefs do you need to change?

What additional skills do you need to develop to be successful and achieve what you want?

For example, if you would benefit from increasing your skills in networking or public speaking, get some help in these areas.

What supports do you need to develop to help you in achieving your challenging goals? Band together with others who support and inspire you during your practice-building efforts.

What daily habits and disciplines will support your productivity and good achievement?

What do you need to change or add to your life to have more energy and vitality?

CONCLUSION

Are You Ready?

The Today's Private Practice approach to earning a living in the psychology and mental health professions is working for many professionals right now. It's about working smarter, not harder.

You can start by joining other Today's Private Practice professionals who are already doing this.

I hope you embrace the challenge of breaking free of managed care and develop a thriving practice that is both rewarding and financially successful.

If you would like to continue the conversation in a supportive environment where questions are answered and more hands-on material is provided, I encourage you to become a Today's Private Practice member.

I invite you to visit www.TodaysPrivatePractice.com and click on the link that says, "I read the book."

Today's Private Practice is about training mental health professionals to earn more money and develop successful practices. On the web site, you will find many resources and practical, often low-cost strategies and how-to ideas you can use to improve your practice immediately and long-term.

Available 24/7, you can access a special introductory offer for professionals at www.TodaysPrivatePractice.com, so you can decide whether this professional development path is for you.

You can also view and register for coaching and practice-building classes and resources at www.WilliamDMorgan.com.

Activate your special introductory offer membership by using the code below at www.TodaysPrivatePractice.com and click on the link that says "I read the book."

Input this code: 569444

We will send you a reminder at the end of the special offer period giving you the opportunity to renew your membership at a monthly fee.

Specifically, the Today's Private Practice membership gives you access to the following:

- One interactive teleseminar per month on a nuts-and-bolts topic concerning building a thriving managed-care free practice.
- Multiple articles and reports on hands-on practice-building strategies and methods, illustrating step-by-step how to accomplish your Today's Private Practice challenges in the Eight Steps.
- Downloadable audio recordings sharing additional crucial information. You can listen to them on your computer or burn them onto a CD to listen to anywhere.

• Group call-in coaching appointments – call in Q&A sessions to answer your unique questions on any of your private practice projects.

• Other perks as part of your membership to Today's Private Practice.

APPENDICES

APPENDIX 1 –
A Working List of Niche Markets

Single mothers
Accountants
Lawyers
Dentists
Human resource professionals
Parents of children with ADHD
Parents of children with Asperger's
or PDD
Police officers
Athletes
Clergy
Divorced fathers
War veterans
Smokers who want to quit
College students
Dating singles
Recently divorced
Career moms
Executives
Family business owners

Couples dealing with infertility
Women business owners
Entrepreneurs
Performers
ADD adults
Cardiac patients
People approaching retirement
Families with Alzheimer's parent
Workaholics
High achievers
Heart patients
Heart transplant recipients
People in debt
Parents of teenagers
College students with learning disabilities
Business and professional people with learning disabilities
Companies in transition or downsizing
Family-owned businesses
Parents of adopted children
People with debilitating chronic illnesses
People who need better social skills
Blended families
recovering alcoholics or other addictions

APPENDIX 2 —
A Working List of Personal Growth/ Skills Building Areas of Felt Need

Stress Management for a specific niche group
Healthy Lifestyle
Parenting/Family
Academic Success
College Success
Divorce Recovery
Co-parenting
Career Transition/Change
Emotional Intelligence
Authentic Happiness (see www.AuthenticHappiness.com)
Resiliency (see www.AdaptivLearning.com)
Relationships
Marriage enrichment
People skills
Work-Life Balance
Achieving Life Balance
Lack of Confidence
Lack of Direction in Life
Better Communication
Conflict Resolution
Unhappy Relationships
People Who Overspend
Weight Management
Bereavement

APPENDIX 3 — A Working List of Traditional (And Some Non-Traditional) Services Not Covered by Managed Care

Psychoeducational Evaluations
Learning Problems
Custody Evaluations
Court-Ordered Evaluations
Forensic Consulting and Evaluations
Business Consulting
Executive Coaching
Personal Coaching
Assisting Troubled Employees
Presenting Workshops
Team Building
Risk Assessments of Students for Schools
Assisting Troubled Students
School Consulting

About the Author

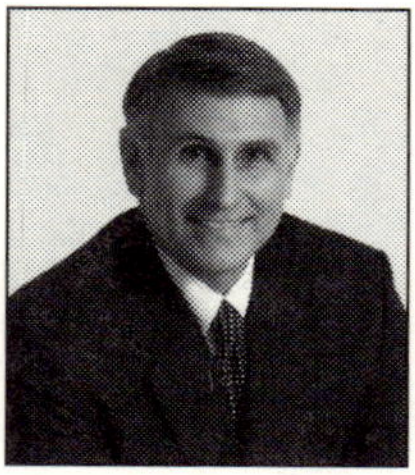

Dr. Bill Morgan is a psychologist in private practice in the Philadelphia area. In addition to his clinical practice, he supports a mix of executives, small business owners and professionals in creating the business, career or lifestyle they wish to achieve through business coaching.

Because of his own experience and dedication to the profession, Bill especially enjoys assisting mental health professionals in designing and building thriving private practices, where therapists and their clients have high levels of satisfaction.

Bill has a doctorate in clinical psychology and is adjunct faculty in the doctoral psychology program at Widener University. He has written a series of professional articles and chapters about the treatment of various problems. He is a popular speaker on issues of personal growth and change.

Bill is a licensed psychologist. He is a member of the American Psychological Association, the Pennsylvania Psychological Association, the International Coach Federation, the Philadelphia Area Coaches Alliance and on the professional advisory board for Chester County CHADD.

GET IN TOUCH

You are welcome to get in touch with Bill and the Today's Private Practice team to:

- Ask a question
- Provide feedback
- Find out about Today's Private Practice workshops
- Receive updates about Today's Private Practice
- Or something else.

By email: info@TodaysPrivatePractice.com

By web site: www.TodaysPrivatePractice.com

By phone: 610.687.7695

By mail: 63 Chestnut Road, Suite Four, Paoli, PA 19301

ACKNOWLEDGEMENTS

All of the charter members of Today's Private Practice

All of the coaching clients I have had the privilege to serve and from whom I've learned

My mentors and coaches

Colleagues who have shared their experiences

The inspiration and concepts I learned through the writings of Andrea Lee (author of Multiple Steams of Coaching Income), Dana Ackley (author of Breaking Free of Managed Care) and C.J. Hayden (author of Get Clients Now).

Jeff Kaplan, fellow psychologist and coach, for his support and inspiration

Dale Morgan for her support and help with the manuscript